They Don't Call It A Vegan Apple

Common Misconceptions About Veganism And Finding Your Way to a Plant-Based Diet

By John Battaglino and Megan Okonsky

Table Of Contents

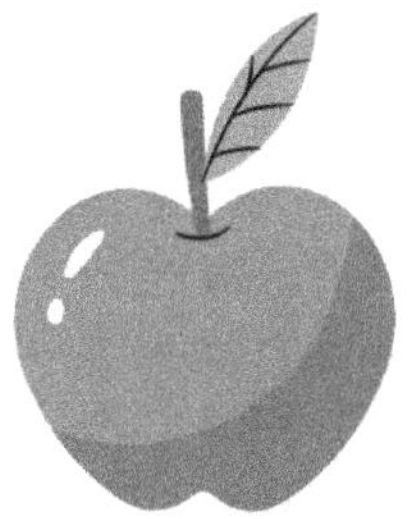

Introduction

What do you think about when you hear the word, "vegan?"

A lot of things might come up: fake cheese, salads, people wearing burlap and protesting for animal rights, you name it. Depending on the people you hang around with or the media you consume, your idea of a "vegan" may have positive or negative connotations.

Veganism has gotten a bad rap over the past few decades. People see veganism as an extreme diet, even tortuous. Vegans are often associated with scare tactics and aggressive messaging that can make others feel uncomfortable. Fortunately, that image is starting to change. Education, media, and even celebrity role models are starting to shine a brighter light on eating a plant-based diet or living a vegan life. How can anyone think that veganism isn't cool when everyone from Beyoncé to Venus Williams to Kyrie Irving is giving it a shot?

You are reading this book for a reason: you are curious about plant-based diets, but don't know where to start. You have questions about veganism, and maybe want some clarity about the misconceptions that you might have heard about vegan diets. You've come to the right place.

Before getting into information about animal rights or the delicious foods that you can enjoy on a vegan diet, let's clear up some of the vocabulary that surrounds this lifestyle, nutrition plan, diet, or whatever you want to call this choice to stick to plant-based foods.

"Vegan" is a relatively new term, although people have chosen to refrain from eating meat or dairy for a long time. In the 1940s, a group of people got together to discuss the lifestyle and choices of non-dairy vegetarians. Donald Watson, and those in the meeting, decided that a new term was needed to identify this new movement. This movement took vegetarianism one step further. Watson decided to shorten "vegetarian" to "vegan," and the Vegan Society was born.

Today, veganism is more than just a choice to refrain from meat and dairy. You don't have to be a member of the Vegan Society to make these choices, either. Veganism typically refers to the choice to refrain from *any* animal byproduct: meat, dairy, eggs, honey, bone char, etc. Vegans may apply this idea not only to their diet, but also to their lifestyle. That means no leather couches, no fur coats, and no cosmetic products that have been tested on animals.

Veganism isn't so cut-and-dry, although some of its loudest proponents may pretend that it is. Not all vegans refrain from honey. Others sit on leather couches. Some raise chickens and eat the eggs that come from these animals.

In this book, we're going to focus on a specific set of choices within veganism: a plant-based diet. "Plant-based" and "vegan" may be used interchangeably, but "plant-based" diets are seen as more flexible than a vegan diet. A person can stick to a plant-based diet and still have a burger occasionally, or eat eggs in the morning.

You will hear one message repeated throughout this book: what you decide to put in your body is your choice. Many back away from a vegan diet because they feel the pressure to take their lifestyle to the extreme. Ignore that pressure. There are many reasons to stick to a plant-based diet, in spite of the misconceptions surrounding plant-based eaters and a vegan lifestyle. We will address these ideas in the first two chapters of the book. But whether or not you decide to eat a plant-based diet should be up to you. You have options for transitioning to this type of diet based on your lifestyle, preferences, and how you prefer to pick up new habits. You also have support when searching for plant-based recipes and learning about what animal byproducts make up your meals. The final two chapters of the book will walk you through the start of your journey into a new diet or lifestyle.

Veganism doesn't have to be extreme. You do not have to give up your favorite foods or sell all of your leather goods in order to improve your life or refine your diet. The choices you make after this book are up to you: your lifestyle, your health, and how you want to approach your diet. So, keep an open mind as you keep reading. Some misconceptions will be cleared up, you will learn something new, and you will have a better understanding of the opportunities that plant-based diets can give you today, tomorrow, and for the rest of your life.

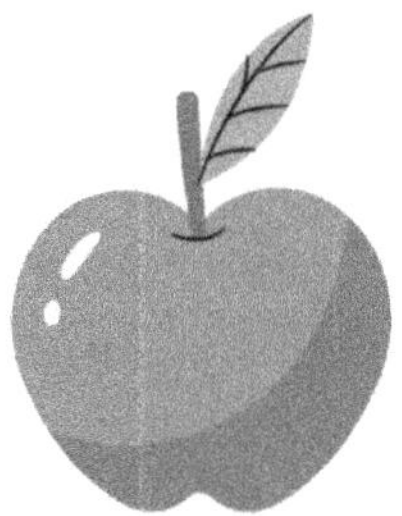

Chapter One: Why Eat Plants, Anyway?

People who have switched to a plant-based diet will likely tell you the effects of their new nutrition plan: they feel great, they have so much energy, they've lost weight, etc. But what about the *causes?* Why do people choose to forgo bacon, fried chicken, and cheese in the first place?

The reality is, there are *so* many reasons to switch to a plant-based diet! We could fill a whole book with the reasons that vegans and plant-based eaters give for adjusting their diet. Instead, we are going to list three categories that explain why most people enjoy a vegan diet: compassion for animals, compassion for the environment, and compassion for their own bodies, minds, and spirits.

The Obvious: Animal Rights

When people think of vegans, they often think of the People for the Ethical Treatment of Animals, or PETA. PETA has a reputation for fighting for animal rights using inflammatory and controversial methods. Some of these methods, including racy ad campaigns and lawsuits alleging that whales were held as "slaves," have turned a lot of people off to PETA's overall mission. One of the stigmas haunting vegans is the association with PETA and other groups that take extreme measures to end the consumption of meat, wearing fur, and other potentially abusive practices.

Does every vegan support PETA? No. Do some vegans choose to eliminate animal products from their diet or lifestyle because they want to support animal rights? Yes.

One can see an obvious connection to vegetarianism and animal rights. Slaughterhouses and factory farms raise animals solely to kill them and meet the demand for meat products around the globe. The World Economic Forum estimates that 50 billion chickens are killed every year for food production. Over 1.5 billion pigs and over 200 million cattle face the same fate. Even more animals die before they are taken to the slaughterhouse due to stress-related activity.

But what does that have to do with cheese production? Eggs? Other animal byproducts? The treatment of cows and other animals to fulfill the demand of dairy and other industries also raises some eyebrows among animal activists. The rapid growth of factory farms often places more animals under unethical conditions.

Cows, for example, can only produce milk while pregnant or giving birth. In order to get the highest yield of milk per cow, cows may be separated from their young or artificially inseminated to keep them producing year-round. Once a cow cannot produce milk, they may be sent to the slaughterhouse. According to the National Humane Education Society, cows in factory farms live for only five years, whereas a cow in a more natural environment can survive for up to 20 years. During this time, cows in factory farms are hooked up to machines that milk them and are kept indoors.

Not all milk or beef products come from factory farms, but over nine million cows currently live on factory farms in the United States. And cows are far from the only animal that undergoes stressful treatment in order to produce foods that we eat everyday. There is a lot more to learn about the unethical treatment of cows, chickens, turkeys, etc. If you are interested in more information about factory farming, check out these documentaries:

- *Death on a Factory Farm*

- *Cowspiracy: The Sustainability Secret*

- *Peaceable Kingdom*

- *Speciesism: The Movie*

(Warning: there is graphic content in many of these movies.)

The Not-So-Obvious: Environmental Reasons

Not all plant-based eaters put animal rights at the top of their list of reasons for cutting meat or dairy out of their diet. Others have a much larger cause in mind: the planet Earth.

Agriculture changed the course of our planet forever. When humans started to farm food, they had a reason and an opportunity to stay put. This resulted in a transition out of a nomadic lifestyle to one that is more sedentary. Homes and towns were built, surrounding the acres of farmland that provides our food.

As our population expanded, so did the need for farmland. Over 40% of the world's land (minus the deserts and areas covered in ice) are used for farming. This farmland, especially in America, has a significant impact on the amount of greenhouse gases we produce. The U.S. EPA believes that 10% of the country's greenhouse gas emissions come from farming, and a significant amount of those emissions come from the gas released by cows who are grazing on farmland. (That's right - cow burps are contributing to climate change.) Impossible Foods, on the other hand, says that their plant-based meat products produce 89% fewer greenhouse gases than beef products.

In order to eat the grass and food that causes cows to let out this gas, they need space to graze. This also has a negative impact. Data collected over recent decades have revealed that 80% of current deforestation rates can be attributed to cattle ranching. Deforestation, especially in areas like the Amazon Rainforest, has a significant impact on the climate. Fewer trees threaten the world's biodiversity and oxygen supply.

Switching to a plant-based diet can severely reduce your carbon footprint, although diet is just one factor that contributes to your impact on the environment.

The Up-To-You: Body, Mind, and Spirit Benefits

Maybe a person's reason for eating a plant-based diet is much smaller than the planet or an entire species. A person could just want to eliminate dairy and meat because they want *themselves* to feel better: physically, mentally, or spiritually.

In the end, there are plenty of reasons for people to make changes to their diet, and they are all valid. Some reasons people eat a plant-based diet include:

- Weight-loss potential

- Inspiration from Beyoncé, Jay-Z, or other celebrities

- The thrill of a challenge

- They personally feel more energized when they are not eating meat

- A vegetarian diet relies too much on dairy, so they decide to eliminate dairy

- Plant-based diets encourage people to eat more fruits and vegetables

- They don't like the taste of meat or cheese

- Religious leaders or doctrine encourage a plant-based diet

You do not *need* a reason to switch up your diet. If you want to eliminate animal byproducts, you have the right to do so. If you want to eat less meat, but don't want to give up cheese board nights with your friends, that's okay. If you want to give veganism a shot for one month, you can always go back later. Do what is right for your body, your values, and your lifestyle.

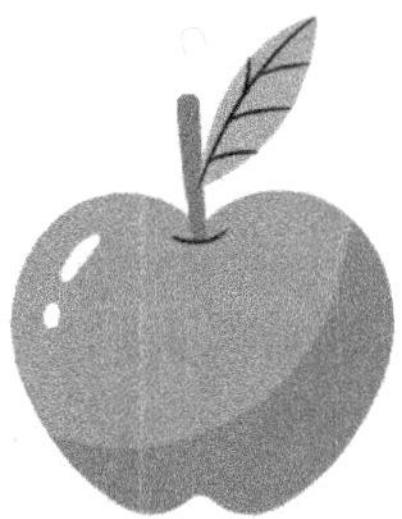

Chapter Two: Why People Aren't Eating Plants - Common Misconceptions about Veganism

For every reason you can think of to go vegan, there is a reason why someone *won't* eliminate animal byproducts from their diet. We all have that one family member who wouldn't even *entertain* the idea of trying a plant-based diet.

Some of these reasons are pretty silly: your uncle might equate eating meat with masculinity. Your mom is hooked on keto and refuses to try any other diet. Your brother tells you that animals were put on this Earth to feed us.

These excuses are easy to brush off, but there are a few arguments that give aspiring vegans pause as they contemplate their diet. Will vegans be missing out on key nutrients by forgoing meat? Will they be miserable? Are they not *actually* vegan if they have a leather couch or sneak a cupcake at a birthday party?

This chapter will address some of the most common misconceptions about veganism. These are common reasons that people use for eating meat or dairy. You might have shared these ideas with friends and family yourself. Don't let these outdated arguments hold you back from trying something new. A vegan diet can be healthy. You can enjoy delicious foods at home, at restaurants, and at fast-food joints. And if you're nervous about "messing up," don't be. The choices you make about your diet may not be identical to another person's, and that's okay. Choosing a plant-based diet is *your* decision.

Misconception #1: Veganism Isn't Healthy

Vegans and vegetarians are asked about protein so often that they tend to have a memorized answer when the subject comes up. Skeptics ask whether a plant-based diet really can provide enough protein to sustain someone. (Others simply state that it cannot.) In addition to misconceptions about protein, skeptics may argue that a vegan cannot get enough Vitamin B in their daily diet.

The truth may be surprising.

Addressing the Protein Myth: According to the CDC, the average adult American woman weighs 170 pounds, while the average adult American male weighs 197 pounds. If the average person sticks to the recommended .36 grams of protein per pound of body weight, they would need 61.2 and 71 grams of protein, respectively. (These numbers will vary based on your body composition and lifestyle - talk to your doctor or a medical professional about the right diet for your body.)

Are you going to reach 61 grams of daily protein by eating bananas (1.3 grams of protein) and onions (1.2 grams of protein) all day? Probably not. But that doesn't mean you can't get daily protein without eating meat.

Lentils are a legume that are popular among plant-based eaters. They can be added to soup, curry, salads, or even tacos. One serving of lentils has 18 grams of protein. Protein patties at Trader Joe's also have 18 grams of protein each - these are made with pea protein and are a great substitute for beef. A cup of chickpeas (often used as a salad topper, or blended into hummus) has a whopping *39* grams of protein. There are plants out there that want to provide you with protein!

If your daily *food* consumption doesn't make the cut, look at your drinks. Plant-based protein powders, like those made with pea protein or hemp protein, are easier to find than ever. One package has up to 20 grams of protein!

Supplementing Your Diet With Vitamins: As with any diet, you might find gaps in certain vitamins and minerals. Vitamin B is typically found in animal byproducts: liver, seafood, eggs, etc. Vegans can find Vitamin B in foods like leafy greens and nutritional yeast, but they might still struggle getting their daily amount. Fortunately, multivitamins are also more common. As the amount of plant-based eaters rise throughout the country, nutrition companies are taking note. Plant-based eaters can choose from over a dozen multivitamins that contain no animal byproducts and help to supplement any gaps that vegans might experience.

Even if you are sticking to meat, dairy, and eggs, your diet will not have *everything* you need by default. Keep track of your daily meals or talk to a nutritionist about what you need in your diet. You have options to find everything you need, from multivitamins to protein shakes to good, old-fashioned fruits and veggies.

Misconception #2: Veganism Isn't Delicious

Cheese tastes pretty good. So does bacon. But so does the Crispy HipCity Ranch sandwich at plant-based fast-casual restaurant HipCityVeg. The Rebel Whopper patties at Burger King are pretty tasty - and completely vegan.

The rising number of plant-based eaters is changing the marketplace. Ten years ago, vegans would have never expected Burger King to have a vegan patty. Today, multiple menu items cater to vegetarians and plant-based eaters. Ten years ago, a plant-based product that looked, tasted, and "bled" like meat seemed impossible. Today, the Impossible Burger (and its rival, the Beyond Burger) are offered at restaurant chains and grocery stores around the country. After +years of demanding more options, you can find delicious and "more authentic" meat *and* dairy replacements wherever you buy your food.

Don't limit your ideas of "vegan food" to rubbery cheese substitutes or something that merely resembles an animal byproduct. You eat vegan food everyday already. No one calls an apple a "vegan apple," but that's just what it is! That banana-mango-orange smoothie you get after pilates? Vegan. The curry you like from the Indian place down the road? Vegan. As you start to examine your diet and the options available to you, you might find that plant-based items are all around. You may also discover new restaurants, meals, or foods that tickle your taste buds. Don't look at a plant-based diet as a limitation. Shift your perspective. You are in a position where you can explore new options and expand your eating horizons. And doesn't that sound delicious?

Misconception #3: It's All or Nothing

Why do activists, nutritionists, and influencers prefer the term "plant-based" over the term "vegan?" "Plant-based" offers more flexibility, both in diet *and* lifestyle. A vegan lifestyle extends beyond a person's diet; a vegan may not wear fur, have a leather couch in their home, or use cosmetic products that have been tested on animals. Not all plant-based eaters make these lifestyle decisions.

A plant-*based* diet may consist exclusively of plants, but non-plant items or byproducts may also slip into a person's diet without coming into conflict with their ethics or the way they choose to structure their diet. An animal activist may feel comfortable eating eggs that came from their neighbor's farm. A vegan may make exceptions for honey or bee pollen. A plant-based eater may choose to adjust their diet when they enter a country or culture where meat is raised, killed, and regarded differently.

You do not have to feel guilty if you decide to reduce, but not completely eliminate, animal byproducts from your diet. If you want to only eat plants during the week, but eat bacon and eggs on Sunday, then only eat plants during the week and eat bacon and eggs on Sunday! If you are switching to a plant-based diet to lose weight, you may keep some foods in your diet that support your health journey. A person who switches to this diet to promote sustainability may make choices based on the carbon footprint of each of their purchases. Your diet affects *your* lifestyle and health. The decision is yours, and yours alone.

Think about your diet and lifestyle choices like the choices you (and others) made during the COVID-19 pandemic. You may have decided to work from home and pull your children from in-person learning, but stay away from the gym or the grocery store. Your neighbor, who doesn't have kids, may have felt safe going to the gym, but reduced their circle of friends. Another neighbor may have felt safe traveling, but only after accessing rapid tests and quarantining. Everyone's lifestyles, mental health, family structure, and access to resources will call for different choices. Do what is best for *you.*

For years, veganism and plant-based diets have felt like a cut-and-dry choice. Either you completely eliminate meat, dairy, and animal byproducts from your diet, or you're "not a real vegan." Get rid of those labels. Remove the stereotypes of a "typical" vegan from your mind. Embrace the new products, brands, and options available to you. Don't let tired misconceptions hold you back from trying out a new diet and potentially changing the way that you eat, drink, and enjoy your life.

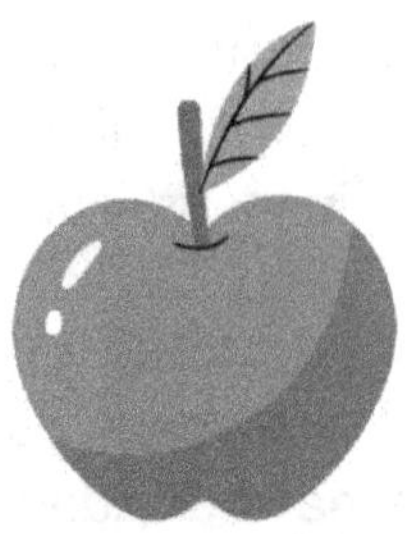

Chapter Three: How to Adopt a Vegan Diet

So you want to switch to a plant-based diet, or start transitioning to a nutrition plan that contains more plants and fewer meals with meat, dairy, or animal byproducts. Amazing! Remember, this is a choice that only you should make (with the help of a nutritionist or medical professional.) The following chapter contains suggestions for ways to make this transition. You may find that going "cold turkey," joining a program, or another strategy works better for you. That's okay! The end goal is what matters: adopting a diet that helps you reach your goals. You are making positive steps to improve your life, and you should be proud of what you're doing each step of the way.

Assess Your Current Diet

Before buying all the tempeh you can find or filling your cabinet with beans, take a look at your current diet. What meals do you like to cook? Do you like to snack throughout the day, or save your calories for larger meals? Are your fruits or veggies more likely to go rotten in your fridge?

Be honest with yourself during this assessment. The best diet transition is an easy one. If you know that you prefer fruit smoothies to raw veggies, going to the store and buying a bunch of produce will only be a waste of money. Instead, budget accordingly so you can make or buy more smoothies and plant-based foods that you already love to eat.

The actual content of your diet may change, but the way that you prepare food, when you eat it, and where you get your food may not have to change all that much. Are you more likely to snack throughout the day? Spend more time looking for plant-based snacks that you can store in your desk.

Assessing your current diet will also help you find replacements to what you're eating now. Do you tend to pop a pizza in the oven on Friday evenings after a long week at work? You don't have to change that routine and make yourself a lentil stew - just search for a plant-based pizza in the frozen aisle. Not *all* of your meals should be frozen, but at least the meals that you tend to eat on the go will have more plant-based ingredients than your previous diet.

As you assess your diet, you may find that you're not getting the nutrients that you need to stay healthy. Consider adding multivitamins or supplements to your shopping list - they can help you in more ways than one as you transition to a new diet.

Start Slow

There is no rulebook for transitioning to an omnivorous diet to something more plant-based. Start slow, and don't feel the pressure to eat 100% vegan right away. Making a slow switch from eating meat to eating more plants can be done by trying the "Meatless Monday" approach, going "food by food," or just taking your diet one meal at a time.

Meatless Monday

One popular way for people to reduce their carbon footprint is trying "Meatless Mondays." They are exactly what they sound like - a full day, each week, without meat (or animal byproducts.) If you're not ready to eliminate all animal products at once, try this approach. Was Meatless Monday a success? Try it again next week - then add on another day of the week. Maybe you eat vegetarian or vegan for two out of seven days for the next couple weeks. That's okay, too.

One Meal At a Time

Alternatively, you could replace meaty breakfasts with something more plant-based. Start by switching up your breakfast. Try an avocado toast with strawberries or sprouts instead of your typical egg sandwich. Or replace the milk in your cereal bowl with almond milk.

If you tend to plan out all of your meals ahead of time, this may be the best strategy for you. Meal prep doesn't have to revolve around grilled chicken or beef bowls. Salads, chickpea dishes, and other options can help you easily grab a plant-based meal on-the-go.

Going Food By Food

Instead of transitioning on a daily or weekly schedule, consider the foods in your diet. Eliminating each meat or dairy item in your diet can help you understand *what* you're having trouble giving up, and also help you see what foods you're not going to miss at all.

Write down a list of all the meats, dairy products, and animal byproducts that you want to eliminate from your diet. (Keep this list handy - as you learn more about how animals are incorporated into everyday foods and food processing, you'll add more ingredients to your list!) Start your transition to a plant-based diet by choosing one or two foods that you want to eliminate from your diet this week or month. These don't all have to be "difficult" foods. Throw yourself a few softballs at first. Sure, you don't eat duck or salmon on a regular basis, but put them on the list anyway. Start your plant-based diet off by keeping duck, salmon, and eggs out of your diet. Indulge yourself in feeling like you're making progress, even if you hadn't planned on eating some of the foods on your list in the first place.

At some points on this journey, you'll find that you don't miss meat at all. At other points, you may struggle. Use this as a way to find out what foods you may "cheat" on once in a blue moon, and what meals you can easily give up or replace with ease.

Interested in learning more about making small changes to your diet or routine in an effective way? Check out the book *Tiny Habits* by Stanford researcher BJ Fogg. The book offers simple solutions to changing your routine and creating habits that enhance your everyday life.

Don't Compare Yourself to Anyone

For some people, starting slow is more effective. You will find that experimentation or trial-and-error sets a strong foundation for a plant-based diet that lasts for years. Other people may find that a "challenge" or quitting overnight works best for them. Don't let another person discourage you, when they live a completely different life or form habits differently. The end goal, whatever it looks like for you, can be achieved in an infinite number of ways. Stick to the methods and strategy that are working best for *you,* and don't be afraid to make changes or show yourself some compassion if you need to switch things up.

Be careful as you scroll through social media. Influencers can provide great recipes and tips for transitioning to a plant-based diet, but these influencers may have been living a vegan lifestyle for years. They may have struggled in the past with sticking to their diet (or they currently struggle, but just refrain from posting about those struggles on their social media accounts.) Don't let anyone you see online make you feel "less than" because you snuck a cupcake at work or had vitamins with gelatin.

Veganism, at its core, is about compassion. Show compassion for yourself by accepting your slip-ups, taking things at your pace, and understanding that you may not have all of the information at your fingertips right now. You have plenty of time to learn about nutrition, animal products, and how your food is made. You also have support. Along your journey, you may encounter judgement, doubt, and skepticism from people in and out of the vegan community. Don't worry about that - people with these feelings are wasting their time worrying about others. Your diet ultimately affects *your* body, not anyone else's. Take the path that is most beneficial to *you,* including finding and interacting with people who want to support you and see you succeed.

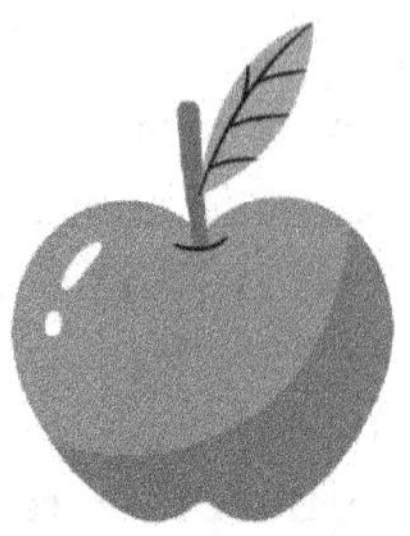

Chapter Four: Where To Find Support

How do we know that there are an infinite amount of ways to live a plant-based lifestyle? There are *so* many people who have made this transition! (This includes people who were born into vegan households and enjoyed a plant-based diet since infancy.) Despite the stereotype of the judgemental vegan or the fierce animal rights activist, you will find a welcoming, compassionate vegan community that is ready and willing to help you make a transition to a more plant-based lifestyle.

No one book will be able to answer all of your questions about a plant-based diet. With more plant-based products coming out every day, you may find more helpful resources in social media groups and online. These four resources are a great place to start if you have questions, need tips, or want to stay updated on news related to veganism and plant-based diets.

Facebook Groups

The *best* resource you can find is other plant-based eaters: friends, coworkers, family members, or anyone who doesn't mind sharing a plate of tempeh for dinner. But this community is not always easy to find in person. Online groups, like forums and Facebook groups, have been a welcome environment for vegans, vegetarians, plant-based eaters, and anyone who may be experimenting with a different nutrition plan.

Facebook groups for plant-based eaters have a variety much like the population of plant-based eaters. Some of these groups cater to "newbies," offering judgment-free zones for people to ask questions as they transition to eating more plants. Other groups focus on recipes, education, or news that may affect the vegan and plant-based communities. You can even join a group of vegan cheese enthusiasts!

Try joining a few of these groups - not all of them may appeal to your goals as a plant-based eater or even what you want to see on your newsfeed. When you do find a group that is interesting, engaging, or helpful, don't be afraid to ask questions! Plant-based eaters love sharing their recipes, tips, and humorous gifs with others. Let these groups be an entry into the larger plant-based community that exists all around the world!

Blogs

If you have a specific question that you can't find in a Facebook group, search for the answer in a blog! Like Facebook groups, there are tons of blogs that help you through your first month as a plant-based eater, review new plant-based products on the market, and give suggestions for making the most out of a plant-based Christmas, Thanksgiving, or other holiday. Many of these websites also have social media following and groups that you can interact with on a daily basis. The amount of online resources within the plant-based community is truly incredible.

Meetups

Prefer to connect offline? Join a meetup for plant-based eaters! No matter where you live, you can probably find a meetup of vegans, vegetarians, or like-minded people that you can connect with and learn from. Look for events on Meetup.com, or ask around at your local farmer's market, health food store, or gym. Vegan restaurants nearby may also offer cooking classes or events specifically catered to plant-based eaters. Yoga studios, holistic health clinics may also be helpful in your search for your local plant-based eaters.

Your local health food store may also host events that cater to the plant-based community. While these events may have been put on hold in 2020, in-person meetups may be making a comeback in the next few years. Talk to the team at your local health food store, gym, or community center about offering meetups and opportunities that bring your local plant-based eaters together.

Barnivore And Other Search Engines

Did you know that your wine may not be vegan-friendly? Egg whites, gelatin, and fish bladders have been used as a filter in winemaking for centuries. These ingredients help to soften the tannins in wine.

Not all winemakers believe in using this technique, but many still do. If you no longer want to drink wine made with this method, you'll have to do some searching the next time you're at the grocery store. Very few wines will advertise whether or not they are vegan-friendly. Fortunately, search engines like Barnivore.com can help you figure out whether your wine (or beer, liquor, or other products) are vegan-friendly.

HappyCow is another popular resource for finding plant-based meals and food items. Leaping Bunny helps you determine whether your favorite brands are cruelty-free. As you continue on your journey, check in with Facebook groups and fellow plant-based eaters to learn about *their* favorite resources.

A Note About Different Resources, Groups, Etc.

As you connect with other vegans, vegetarians, and plant-based eaters, remember that your nutrition plan is *your* choice. Facebook groups may have rules against judgement, bias, or harsh words against people who eat dairy or meat items. They may not, and the culture within certain groups (online or off) may not feel so welcoming. Do not be discouraged. For every person who may pass judgement, there is another person who opens their arms to people who eat the occasional strip of bacon or host wine and cheese parties. If you haven't found a group of resources that support your goals, you just have to search a little longer.

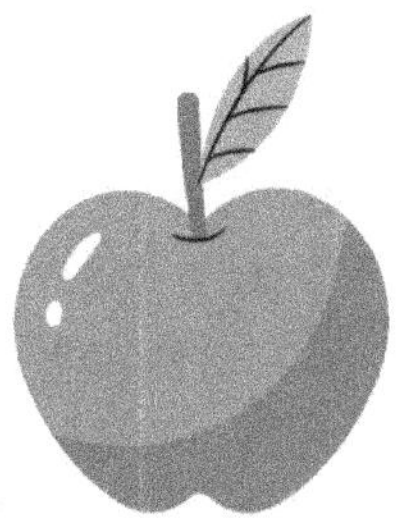

Ready, Set, Eat!

When is the best time to start the transition into a plant-based diet? Right now! That transition will look different for everyone. Your next meal may be a tempeh sandwich, a salad, or a slice of pizza and "cheese" fries from the vegan restaurant down the street. That transition may also look like switching out dark meat for white meat, adding a green smoothie to your meal, or forgoing the request to leave the tomato and lettuce *off* your burger. All of these meals are great choices, and none make you a "better" or "worse" plant-based eater.

The misconceptions about vegans come from many places: movies, televisions, judgemental relatives, you name it. In the past, they have held many people back from trying out a diet that contains no meat or dairy. "Vegan food" is passed up for barbeque, even when that "vegan food" is a healthy salad and protein that you could find on any menu around the country.

Now that you've learned about veganism, its origins, and *why* people take on a plant-based diet, I hope your mind is more open to experimenting with your nutrition and making choices that are right for *you.* Maybe you want to lose a little weight, challenge yourself to try new foods, or just be like your friends who have made the switch. Great! Assess your diet, find some places to make changes, and know that you have many people supporting you. You may just discover something great that helps you, animals, and the planet for many years to come.